AMAZING HOLIDAY APPETIZER RECIPES.

26 Healthy Recipes For Healthy Living.

JOLLY SPARK

TABLE OF CONTENT

1. <u>ROASTED BERRY CREAM CHEESE SPREAD</u>

This roasted berry cream cheese spread is the perfect topping to your morning bagel or as a delicious fruit dip. Ready in under 30 minutes and packed full of sweet berry flavor. You'll want to this spread on everything!

yield: 2 cups cream cheese spread

prep time: 10 minutes
cook time: 15 minutes
total time: 25 minutes

Ingredients:
1/2 cup quartered strawberries
1/2 cup blueberries
1-2 tablespoons dark brown sugar
16 ounces' cream cheese, room temperature

Directions:
Preheat oven to 425 degrees and line a rimmed baking sheet with parchment paper.
Add strawberries and blueberries to the prepared baking sheet and sprinkle with dark brown sugar. Toss to combine. Roast for about 15 minutes or until the berries are slightly soft. Remove from the oven and let cool.
Once the berries are cool (it won't take too long) add cream cheese to the bowl of an electric mixer and beat for a minute just to get it fluffy. Add in the berries and mix for a few minutes or until the berries are fully combined into the cream cheese. Make sure to stop once to scrape down the sides. Keep the roasted berry cream cheese spread in the refrigerator until ready to use.

2. AVOCADO & SHRIMP APPETIZERS

Preparation Time: 10 min

Ingredients:
1. 14 Cocktail Shrimp – Fully Cooked, Deveined etc.
2. 1 Avocado
3. 14 Cherry Tomatoes
4. Red Pepper Flakes
5. Salt
6. Black Pepper
7. Chipotle Pepper

Instructions:
1. Thaw your shrimp. You can do this by putting them in the fridge overnight, or rinsing them in hot water.
2. Then prepare the avocado. Slice the avocado into small chunks and set aside. When everything is prepared, use toothpicks to put the appetizers together.
3. Put the tomato, avocado, and shrimp on your toothpick like little skewers.
4. Place them all on a serving tray.
5. Top with a pinch of salt, red pepper flakes, black pepper, and chipotle pepper. This gives it a little bit of heat and flavor, but not too much to overpower the other flavors. Plus, it gives it some more color! You can serve with cocktail sauce on the side, or not. We think it's great without but it's completely up to you.

3. APPETIZER «FRENCH»

Ingredients:
- Proteins of egg — 4 pcs.
- Cheese—200g.
- Wheat flour — 1 tbsp
- Vegetable oil — for deep frying.
- Parsley.
- Salt and ground black pepper to taste.

Preparation:
1. Proteins will beat into a soft, adding a little grated cheese. The resulting mass salt and pepper.
2. Make small balls, roll them in flour and fry in hot oil. When the balls will increase in volume, remove them with a slotted spoon from the pan and dry. Serves, put on a warmed platter and sprinkle with parsley.

4. MINI PIZZA APPETIZERS

Preparation time 10 mins
Cook time 20 mins
Total time 30 mins
Serves: 6

Ingredients:
- 6 small Portobello mushroom caps
- 2 tbs. olive oil
- Salt to taste
- ½ cup pizza sauce
- ¾ cup grated mozzarella
- ½ cup cherry tomatoes
- 1 tbs. fresh basil

Instructions:
1. Preheat the oven to 425 degrees.
2. Brush the Portobello mushrooms with olive oil, then sprinkle with salt to taste. Place the mushrooms in a single layer on a wire rack on top of a baking sheet. Cook in the 425 degrees' oven for 5 to 10 minutes, or until they're beginning to get tender. (The wire rack keeps the mushrooms from getting soggy. Timing will vary according to the size of the mushrooms.)
3. Remove the baking sheet from the oven and top the mushrooms with pizza sauce, cheese, and cherry tomatoes.
4. Return the mushrooms to the oven and bake for another 8 to 10 minutes, or until the cheese is melted. Sprinkle with fresh basil and serve.

5. ASIAN TERIYAKI MEATBALL APPETIZERS

The combination of beef and pork in the meatballs adds an extra degree of tenderness and flavor to these awesome Asian teriyaki meatball appetizers. These easy to make bite-sized babes are oven-baked then drenched in a special teriyaki sauce that puts a delicious glaze on them.

Ingredients:
- 1-pound ground beef
- 1-pound ground pork
- ½ cup Panko breadcrumbs
- 2 large egg yolks
- 1 tablespoon tahini sauce
- 2 green onions, thinly sliced
- 2 cloves garlic, grated
- 2 tablespoon freshly grated ginger
- 1 tablespoon soy sauce
- 1 teaspoon Chinese five-spice powder
- ½ teaspoon white pepper
- Sesame seeds and snipped chives or green onion tops for garnish
- Wooden picks for serving

For the teriyaki sauce
- 1 tablespoon cornstarch
- ¼ cup soy sauce
- 2 tablespoons brown sugar, packed
- 1 tablespoon grated fresh ginger root
- 1 fresh garlic clove, grated
- 2 tablespoons hoisin sauce
- 2 tablespoons honey

Instructions:

1. Preheat the oven to 400°F Spray a wire rack with cooking spray set over a baking sheet that has been lined with aluminum foil. (For easy clean-up)

2. In a large bowl, combine ground beef, ground pork, bread crumbs, egg yolks, tahini, green onions, garlic, ginger, soy sauce, five-spice powder and white pepper. Stir together just until well combined; do not over-mix or the meatballs will become tough. Use a small 1 tablespoon size scoop to portion the meat and roll into approximately 60 meatballs.

3. Place meatballs onto prepared baking sheet and bake until golden brown and cooked through, about 20-25 minutes. While the meatballs are baking, make the sauce.

To Make the Teriyaki Sauce:

1. In a small dish, make a slurry of the cornstarch by whisking it with ¼ cup water. Reserve.

2. In a saucepan over medium heat, add soy sauce, brown sugar, grated ginger root, grated garlic, hoisin sauce, honey and 1 cup water, bring to a simmer. Whisk in cornstarch mixture until thickened enough to coat the back of a spoon, about 2 minutes. Remove from the heat and add the cooked meatballs, turning to coat each one.

3. Transfer the meatballs to a serving plate, garnish with sesame seeds and snipped green scallions or chives. Add a pick to each meatball and serve.

6. SALMON TORTILLA APPETIZERS

Ingredients:
- 15 oz Salmon, canned; flaked
- 8 oz Cream cheese; softened
- 4 tb Salsa; mild or medium
- 2 tb Fresh parsley
- 1 tea poons Cilantro
- 1/4 ts Ground cumin; optional
- 8 Flour tortillas; 8 inch

Original recipe makes 48 Servings

Preparation:
Drain salmon and remove any bones. In a small bowl combine salmon, cream cheese, salsa, parsley and cilantro. Add cumin if desired. Spread about 2 tablespoons mixture over each tortilla. Roll each tortilla up tightly and wrap individually with plastic wrap. Refrigerate 2-3 hours; slice each tortilla into bite-size pieces. Yield: About 48 appetizers.

7. <u>ROASTED STRAWBERRIES BRIE APPETIZER</u>

Yield: 6-8
Preparation time: 15 minutes
Cook time: 20 minutes
Total time: 35 minutes

If you don't have a baker for the Brie, you can place the round on a parchment-lined baking sheet.

Ingredients:
- 8 oz. strawberries, quartered, plus extra for garnish
- 2 Tbsp. maple syrup
- 1 Tbsp. olive oil
- Kosher salt
- 1 (13.4 ounce) Brie cheese round Crackers.

Directions:
1. Preheat oven to 400 degrees.
2. Toss strawberries in maple syrup, olive oil, and salt. Place on a parchment-lined baking sheet and bake at 400 degrees for 20 minutes, until juicy and softened.
3. Remove Brie from wrapper and place in a small round baker (or a parchment-lined baking sheet). Bake for 20 minutes, or until crust is brown.
4. Allow to cool for 3 minutes. Take a knife and slice off the top of the Brie, cutting down to remove the top and about 1/2" of the Brie. Top with warm roasted strawberries (with sauce); place the lid back on top.
5. Serve with toasted bread or crackers!

8. APPETIZER WITH PINEAPPLE

Ingredients:
Canned pineapples — Bank 1.
Cheese durum — 100 g.
Chicken Eggs — 2.
Salad «Iceberg» — 1 bunch.
Mayonnaise home — 1 table spoon.

Preparation:
- Remove the pineapple rings from a jar, put them on a dish. Tear off pieces of lettuce and cover the hole of the pineapple, then to the filling does not fall out.
- For the filling: combine chopped into large cubes hard-boiled eggs, cheese and crab sticks. Fill it all with mayonnaise.
- Put the filling on pineapple.

9. HOT DOG PINEAPPLE KABOBS

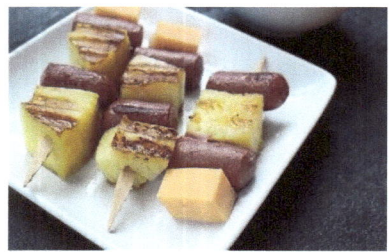

Preparation time: 10 mins
Cook time: 10 mins
Total time: 20 mins

Recipe type: Main Dish
Serves: 2 servings

Ingredients
- 4 Simple Truth Uncured Beef Hot Dogs
- 16 pineapple chunks
- 8 cheddar cheese cubes
- 4 skewers
- Optional: BBQ sauce or ketchup for dipping

Instructions
1. Skewer hot dog pieces and pineapple chunks alternately onto 4 skewers.
2. Spray grill pan or grill with nonstick spray and bring to medium-high heat.
3. Add skewers and cook 3 to 4 minutes. Flip, and cook another 3 to 4 minutes.
4. Once cool enough to handle, pull the food off the grill and add cheese to each end of the skewer.
5. Eat with your favorite hot dog dipping sauce!

10.   GRILLED POTATO KABOBS

To ensure that potatoes are cooked on the inside before they are fully grilled on the outside, first partially cook them in the microwave. You need to only grill them until they are crisp and golden brown.

Serves: Makes 6 servings.
Preparation time: 10mins.
Cooking time: 20mins.

Ingredients:
*   2 pounds unpeeled Yukon Gold potatoes, scrubbed
*   6 wooden skewers
*   3 tablespoons
*   2 tablespoons vegetable oil

Directions
*   Cut potatoes into 1 1/2-inch cubes. Tread onto skewers, leaving some space in between each potato cube.
*   Microwave kabobs on HIGH 8 to 10 minutes or until potatoes are nearly tender. Brush with oil and sprinkle with Barbecue Seasoning.
*   Grill over medium-high heat 8 to 10 minutes or until potatoes are tender and golden brown, turning occasionally.

Nutrition information
(Amount per serving)
*   Calories: 173Cholesterol: 0mg
*   Sodium: 445mgProtein: 3g
*   Total Fat: 5gFiber: 4g
*   Carbohydrate: 29g

11. SOUTHWESTERN PORK KABOBS

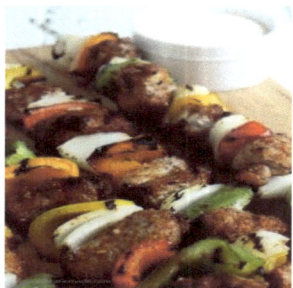

Preparation time: 10 mins
Cook time: 10 mins
Total time: 20 mins

Add a little kick to your grill! These Southwestern Pork Kabobs are full of flavor, easy enough for a weeknight meal but special enough to serve at a party!

Recipe type: Grilling
Serves: serves 4

Ingredients

- 4 Pork Chops - cut into 1 inch cubes
- 4 tablespoons taco seasoning
- ½ large onion - peeled and cut into chunks
- ½ each red, yellow, orange and green peppers - cleaned and cut into chunks
-

Instructions

1. Cut pork and vegetables
2. Place pork in a large plastic reseal-able bag, add taco seasoning and shake to coat
3. Thread pork and vegetables onto skewer

4. Note - if using wooden skewers, they need to soak in water at least 20 minutes before using
5. Grill kabobs over medium-high heat turning occasionally
6. Cook for about 10 minutes

12. GREEN BALSAMIC BEEF KABOBS

Prep Time: 4 hours
Cook Time: 10 minutes
Total Time: 4 hours, 10 minutes
Yield: 4 kabobs
1 kabob

Ingredients
- 1 cup packed fresh parsley
- 1/4 cup extra virgin olive oil
- 1/4 cup coconut amino
- 2 Tb balsamic vinegar
- 2 lbs sirloin or chuck beef, cut into 2 inch cubes
- 2-3 medium red onions, quartered
- 1/2 pound mushrooms (or enough for 3-4 mushrooms per kabob)

Instructions
1. In a high-powered blender or food processor, combine the first four ingredients. Blend until smooth - the marinade will be a lovely green color. Add the beef cubes to a large shallow dish and pour the marinade overtop. Cover and refrigerate for at least 4 hours or overnight.

2. When you're ready to make the kabobs, turn on the grill and preheat to medium-high (400-500 degrees F).

3. Remove the marinated beef from the fridge and prepare to assemble the kabobs. Thread one cube of beef on the skewer, then a mushroom, then a chunk of onion (plus any additional veggies). Continue until skewer is full and repeat with remaining skewers. This recipe made 4 hefty kabobs for me, but you may have more depending on how heavily you load up your skewers or if you add veggies. If you'd like, you can brush the leftover marinade on the veggies, but it's not required.

4. Grill the kabobs on all 4 sides for roughly 2 1/2 minutes on each side.

13. <u>AVOCADO HUMMUS</u>

Ingredients
- 1 can chickpeas
- 1 ripe avocado
- 1 tbsp tahini
- 2 garlic cloves

Instructions
1. Place all ingredients in a food processor and process until smooth and creamy!
2. Garnish with olive oil, and some paprika.
   Pineapple Chicken Kabobs Recipe

14.   SWEET PINEAPPLE KABOB

Serves: about 10 kabobs

Ingredients
- 1 fresh pineapple
- 1 and ½ lbs boneless skinless chicken breast
- 1 red onion
- 1 medium red bell pepper
- 1 medium yellow or orange bell pepper

For the marinade:
- ¼ cup pineapple juice (I got exactly that much after coring fresh pineapple - see note)
- 3 Tablespoons olive oil
- 2 teaspoons apple cider vinegar or lemon juice
- 2 garlic cloves, grated
- ⅓ cup packed light brown sugar
- 3 Tablespoons low-sodium soy sauce
- ½ teaspoon salt
- ¼ teaspoon black pepper

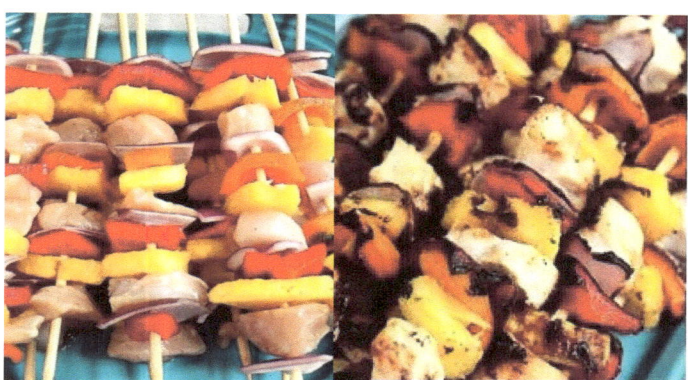

Instructions

1. Core pineapple and pour the juice into a small bowl.
2. To make marinade: combine all ingredients with pineapple juice in small bowl. Mix well. Set aside.
3. Cut chicken into bite size pieces. Place in a bowl, Pour half of the marinade over chicken. Cover and refrigerate for at least 30 minutes. Keep the remaining marinade for glazing.
4. Prepare pineapple, peppers and onion by cutting into fairly the same size pieces (see post photos for reference).
5. Start your grill.
6. Skewer chicken (discard the marinade it was chilling in), pineapple and veggies onto bamboo skewers. Use three to four pieces of chicken per kabob. When piercing the pineapple pieces, go slow to prevent breaking.
7. Grill, brushing with remaining marinade once, until the chicken is done (it should reach the internal temperature of 165 degrees F.

15. BACON CHEESEBURGER MEATBALLS ARE THE PERFECT LOW-CARB APPETIZER

Here's how to whip up a batch yourself.
Ingredients:
- Package of pre-cooked frozen meatballs
- American Cheese, cut in small pieces
- Pre-Cooked Bacon slices, cut in small pieces
- Iceberg Lettuce, cut into small pieces
- Grape Tomatoes, cut in half

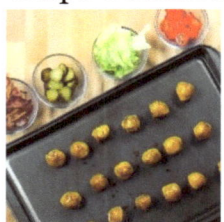 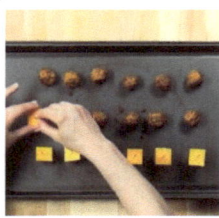 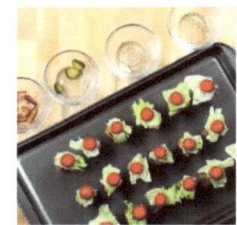

Directions:

1. Bake up as many meatballs as you desire, following the package instructions.
2. Meanwhile: cut small pieces of American cheese to melt on top when meatballs are baked.
3. "Stack" your desired toppings on toothpicks. I used a piece of bacon, a small piece of ice berg lettuce and a half grape tomato.
4. When the baking time is up, top each meatball with a small slice of cheese, place back in the oven for a couple of minutes more to let the cheese melt.
5. Poke the already stacked skewer into the meatball, plate and serve.
6. Serve with ketchup, mayo and mustard dipping "sauce" if desired.

16. LEMON WALNUT ROASTED RED PEPPER DIP

Preparation Time: 15 minutes
Yield: 3 cups

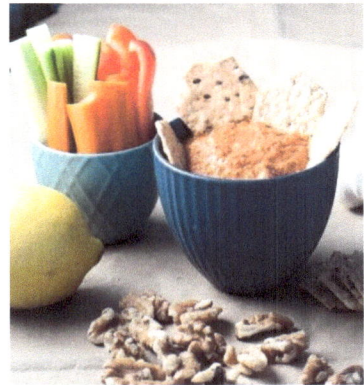

Ingredients

- 16 oz. jar of roasted red peppers (drain well)
- 1 c. walnuts
- juice from 1/2 of a lemon
- 2 garlic cloves
- 1 tsp. cumin
- 1 tsp. corriander
- 2-3 T. extra virgin olive oil
- salt and pepper
- *optional: red pepper flakes, chili powder

Instructions

1. Put all ingredients except olive oil in food processor.
2. Pulse until well combined.
3. Scrape down sides.
4. Add olive oil while running.

vegan, paleo, and gluten free!

17. SALMON TORTILLA APPETIZERS

Ingredients:

- 15 oz **Salmon**, canned; flaked
- 8 oz **Cream cheese**; softened
- 4 tb Salsa; mild or medium
- 2 tb Fresh **parsley**
- 1 ts **Cilantro**
- 1/4 ts Ground **cumin**; optional
- 8 Flour **tortilla**s; 8 inch
- Original recipe makes 48 Servings

Preparation:

Drain salmon and remove any bones. In a small bowl combine salmon, cream cheese, salsa, parsley and cilantro. Add cumin if desired. Spread about 2 tablespoons mixture over each tortilla. Roll each tortilla up tightly and wrap individually with plastic wrap. Refrigerate 2-3 hours; slice each tortilla into bite-size pieces. Yield: About 48 appetizers.

18. ROASTED STRAWBERRIES BRIE APPETIZER

Yield: *6-8*
Prep time: *15 minutes*
Cook time: *20 minutes*
Total time: *35 minutes*

Ingredients:
- 8 oz. strawberries, quartered, plus extra for garnish
- 2 Tbsp. maple syrup
- 1 Tbsp. olive oil
- Kosher salt
- 1 (13.4 ounce) Brie cheese round Crackers

Directions:
1. Preheat oven to 400 degrees.
2. Toss strawberries in maple syrup, olive oil, and salt. Place on a parchment-lined baking sheet and bake at 400 degrees for 20 minutes, until juicy and softened.
3. Remove Brie from wrapper and place in a small round baker (or a parchment-lined baking sheet). Bake for 20 minutes, or until crust is brown.
4. Allow to cool for 3 minutes. Take a knife and slice off the top of the Brie, cutting down to remove the top and about 1/2" of the Brie. Top with warm roasted strawberries (with sauce); place the lid back on top.
5. Serve with toasted bread or crackers!

If you don't have a baker for the Brie, you can place the round on a parchment-lined baking sheet.

19. <u>BABA GHANOUSH HUMMUS</u>

Combine two of the best dip recipes to make Baba Ghanoush Hummus! Full of deep, smoky, and roasted flavors, this condiment will seem like a meal! Gluten-free, vegan, and nut-free, with eggplant and chickpeas, you'll get your healthy veggies and protein in one dip!

Recipe type: Condiment, Snack
Cuisine: Middle Eastern
Serves: 3 Cups

Ingredients:
- 2 Cups Cooked Chickpeas
- 1½ Cups Roasted Eggplant (about 1 medium sized)
- 1 TB Fresh Chopped Cilantro (more for topping)
- 1 TB Harissa
- 1 TB Tahini
- 1 Tsp Lemon Juice
- ½ Tea spoon Smoked Paprika
- ½ Tea spoon Minced Garlic
- ½ Tea spoon Onion Powder
- ¼ Tea spoon Cumin
- Water (as needed to help blend)
-

Instructions:
1. To roast the eggplant, preheat the oven to 450 F. Cut the eggplant top off, then cut the eggplant in half lengthwise. Make cuts in a cross-stitch pattern, through the flesh for easy scooping. Roast in the oven on a baking sheet for 20-30 minutes until very soft. Remove and let cool.

2. In a large food processor, combine all ingredients. For the eggplant either scoop out all the flesh and add to the processor, or like I did, just chop it up and include the skin.

3. Blend the mixture until creamy smooth, adding a bit of water if necessary.

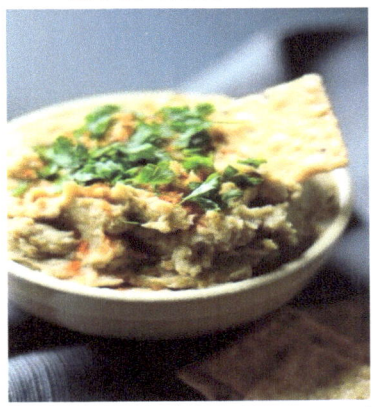

Ah, the glorious taste of roasted and smokey eggplant with the aromas of cumin and harissa! It truly is just decadent to the senses! I do feel like this could be a meal within itself! Veggies, plant-protein and carbs, a little spice to jazz it up, and healthy fats from the harissa and tahini! So for now, eat this as a dip with some crackers or veggies, spread it on a sandwich

20. **VEGAN CRAB CAKES WITH AVOCADO**

Ingredients
- 1 can hearts of palm, diced
- 1/2 avocado, mashed
- 1/4 cup diced red pepper
- 1/4 cup diced red onion
- 2 teaspoons old bay seasoning
- 1 cup cooked quinoa
- 1/4 cup quinoa flour
- salt, to taste
- For the sauce:
- 1/4 avocado,
- 1 tablespoon tahini
- 1 tablespoon extra-virgin olive oil
- 1 tablespoon lemon juice
- salt to taste

Instructions
1. In a bowl combine the crab cake ingredients, hearts of palm, 1/2 mashed avocado, red pepper, red onion, old bay, cook quinoa and salt to taste. Mix. Add quinoa flour. Mix. Form into 6-8 round crab cakes and freeze for 15-20 minutes.
2. In a blender combine the sauce ingredients, 1/4 avocado, tahini, olive oil, lemon juice and salt to taste.
3. Heat 1-2 tablespoons olive oil over medium heat in a pan. Pan fry the patties until browned on each side.

Content: Calories-155cal, Fat-12g, Carbs-12g, Protein-3g.

21.   SWEET BBQ CHICKEN KABOBS

Ingredients

- 1 lb. (450 g) boneless skinless chicken breasts, cut into 1-1/2-inch pieces
- 2 cups fresh pineapple chunks (1-1/2 inch)
- 1 each red and green pepper, cut into 1-1/2-inch chunks
- 1/2 cup BBQ Sauce
- 3 Tbsp. frozen orange juice concentrate, thawed

Instructions

1. Heat barbecue to medium-high heat.
2. Thread chicken alternately with pineapple and peppers onto 8 long wooden skewers, using 2 skewers placed side-by-side for each kabob.
3. Mix remaining ingredients. Reserve half the sauce; brush remaining sauce onto kabobs.
4. Grill 8 to 10 min. or until chicken is done, turning and brushing occasionally with reserved sauce.

22. AMAZING CHEESE BALLS

Ingredients:
- 500g of mozzarella or hard cheese
- 3 tbsp. l. grated parmesan cheese
- 1 egg
- 100 g flour
- 0,5 h. L. oregano
- breadcrumbs
- vegetable oil for frying

Preparation:
Mix the grated cheese or mozzarella, egg and parmesan. Add the flour mixture and oregano. Prepare smooth soft testa. Skatayte small balls of cheese testa. Obvalyayte them in breadcrumbs and store up to 30 minutes in holodilnik. Raskalite oil in a frying pan and fry the balls until golden brown. Drain on paper polotentse.Podavayte to the table. Ready-made cheese balls can be dipped in ketchup, mustard or any other sauce of your choice.

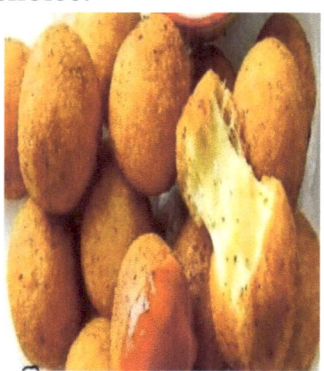

23. __GUACAMOLE__

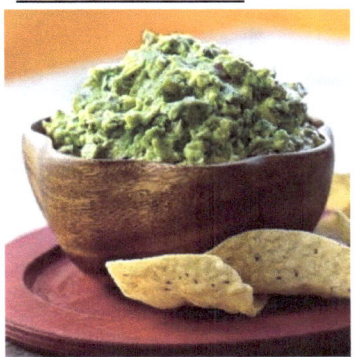

Ingredients:
- 5 ripe avocados
- 2 tablespoons finely chopped red onion
- 2 tablespoons fresh lime juice
- 1/2 medium jalapeño pepper, seeded and chopped
- 1 garlic clove, pressed
- 3/4 teaspoon salt
- Tortilla chips

Direction:
Cut avocados in half. Scoop pulp into a bowl, and mash with a potato masher or fork until slightly chunky. Stir in chopped red onion and next 4 ingredients. Cover with plastic wrap, allowing wrap to touch mixture, and let stand at room temperature 30 minutes. Serve guacamole with tortilla chips.

Cilantro Guacamole: Mash avocado, and stir in ingredients as directed. Stir in 3 Tbsp. chopped fresh cilantro and an additional 1 Tbsp. lime juice. Cover mixture, and let stand at room temperature 30 minutes.

While storing in the refrigerator, keep your guacamole from changing color by placing a layer of plastic wrap directly on the surface of the mixture.

24. ROASTED EDAMAME...PERFECT FOR A LIGHT APPETIZER OR SNACK

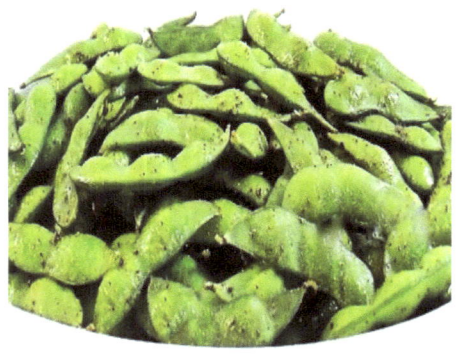

What a great discovery for those of us who like to munch! Packed with protein and fibre, these little green gems make a fun, satisfying, skinny snack or appetizer. Normally boiled, I found they're supremely tasty when roasted. I've generously seasoned them before popping in the oven. Be sure to make oodles of these wonder veggies because they take minutes to prep before roasting and disappear as quickly...

Preparatory Time: 5 minutes

Bake Time: 25 minutes

Ingredients

- 2 teaspoons olive oil
- ½ teaspoon chili powder
- ¼ teaspoon onion powder
- ¼ teaspoon ground cumin
- ⅛ teaspoon paprika
- 1-pound bag frozen edamame (in pods), thawed
- ½ teaspoon salt
- Fresh ground pepper

Instructions

1. Preheat oven to 375 degrees.
2. In a small bowl, stir together the olive oil, chili powder, onion powder, cumin, and paprika.
3. Spread the thawed edamame on a baking pan. Drizzle the olive oil mixture over the top and toss to coat. Arrange edamame in a single layer on the baking pan.
4. Roast uncovered in oven for about 12 to 15 minutes until they start to brown. Season with more salt and pepper, if desired
5. Serve warm. Roasted Edamame can be prepared a day in advance, refrigerated and warmed before serving.
6. Makes 6 servings

Food Fact

Edamame is the Japanese name for green soybeans. These fresh soybeans are picked when they're fully grown but before they become completely mature. To eat, pop the pods and shell them as you would peanuts.

Healthy Benefit

Edamame (soybeans) have many benefits. They're extremely high in protein and fiber, provide useful amounts of B vitamins, significant calcium and a little zinc. Some research has indicated that a soybean rich diet may help prevent or slow the spread of breast cancer.

25. HOT APPETIZER «ABOUT THE CHICKEN»

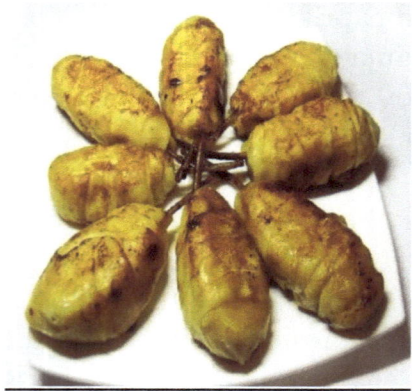

Ingredients for the dough:
-250g of flour
-kefir — 0.75 cups — 1 Cup (depends on flour)
-soda — 1/2 tea spoon of lies.
-salt on the tip of a knife
-500g chicken meat (+1луковица, salt, black pepper to taste)
-1 nayka straw salt
-vegetable oil for frying

Preparation:

1. From yogurt, soda, salt and flour knead the dough (should be soft, not stick to hands).
2. Roll the dough into a thickness of 1 mm and cut into strips of width 3 see
3. Minced knead well, even a little to leave on the table, well-kept, and not broken up.
4. Take a straw, a little meat to stick to the edge of the straw.
5. Then the test strip to obratiti around the stuffing, starting from the middle of the straw and get «chicken leg»
6. In a pan pour oil enough to cover the half of the «legs», it is about 1-1,5 cm, Heat the oil and fry there «legs» to Browning.

Bon appetite!

26. NEW YEAR: APPETIZER IDEAS PARMESAN BITES

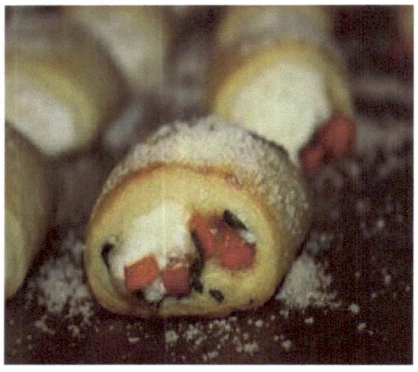

Ingredients:

8 oz of cream cheese, softened, 1 c. grated parmesan cheese, divided, 2 (8 oz) cans of crescent rolls, 1 c. of chopped red pepper, 1/4 c. fresh parsley.

*You can substitute the fresh peppers for drained, roasted red peppers, pepperonni etc

Instructions:

1. Beat Cream cheese, and 3/4 cup of parmesan cheese.

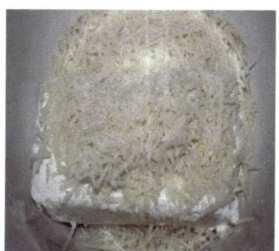

2. Chop parsley and red pepper.

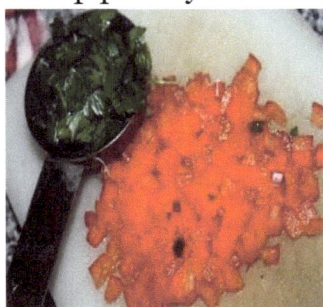

3. Roll out dough, break apart pairs of crescent triangles, and press seams to make a rectangle. Place three T of cheese mix, and sprinkle with peppers and parsley.

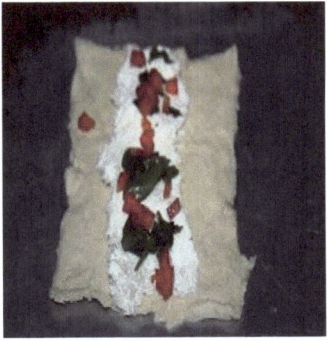

4. Fold and press edges together, and then slice into 4 equal pieces. Sprinkle with the last 1/4 of parmesan (I switched to the bottled kind at this point.... I just like it better as a topping, but do whatever floats our cheese boat).

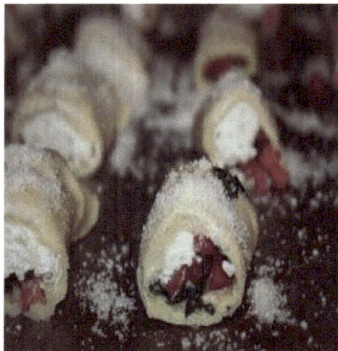

5. Bake at 350 for 13-15 minutes.

32 servings total.

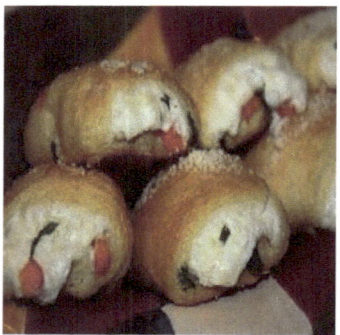

You may be bothered to ask why I said "cut these into 4 pieces" but later said it makes 32 pieces. What I actually mean is that There are eight triangles in a can of crescents. Each set of two triangles -one rectangle-make four pieces. That's 16 pieces per can- 32 pieces for the entire recipe which calls for two cans.

This recipe is my favorite of all. It is best for party...

www.ingramcontent.com/pod-product-compliance
Lightning Source LLC
Chambersburg PA
CBHW050757290526
45792CB00008B/2223